Lose Weight

Lose Weight Permanently

Effective Strategies on How to Lose Weight Easily and Permanently

Introduction

<u>Don't let the hardships you experience in any diet stop you from losing weight with ease. With the strategies that this book discusses, losing weight and keeping it off shouldn't be such an energy, emotional and willpower sucking feat!</u>

Even though most of us hate the idea of waking up early each morning to go for a workout, **the satisfaction that comes with effective weight control is often worth the trouble/effort**. Weight loss or management can be complex especially when your efforts don't seem to produce any tangible results. Setting weight goals is the first step attaining your dream weight.

However, it is likely that **<u>you may lose the motivation to continue with trying to lose weight either because you don't see results as fast as you expect or simply because you don't see any direct benefits that come with losing weight</u>**.

In this book, I discuss some **of the strategies you can use to shed off those extra kilos/pounds and still maintain the motivation to continue practicing habits meant to help you manage your weight**.

Everyone is different; **so do the strategies that work for different people. Having seen people who have battled weight problems in the past**, I have captured all the strategies that each of them used to deal with their problem.

In this book, you will learn:

- How to adjust your food diary to help you lose weight effectively

- **How to take charge of your workouts to make weight loss an effortless affair**

- How to infuse passion in your workouts for effortless weight loss

- **How to leverage on external factors to make weight loss easier**

- And much, much more!

If you are looking for a weight loss approach that works, this book offers a clear and easy to follow approach.

Let's begin!

I hope you enjoy it!

Table of Contents

Adjust Your Food Diary

Don't Starve Yourself As A Way To Fight Obesity

While some people think that reducing intake of food can be a great way to fight obesity, studies show that this can be a slow way of killing yourself. Each of us knows that the body acts as a storage for nutrients and fats among other essential components that are controlled by nutrition in form of vitamin, food, beverages and mineral supplements. Many of us who have studied the body, its components and operations know that when it lacks nutritional components, it starts using the stored reserves so as to maintain its operation at equilibrium.

If the body keeps on consuming the stored nutrients, a quick drop in metabolism is observed which means the body would have to protect its insulating fats by consuming muscle stores as a way to recover from the lack of calorie intake. Once your body metabolism drops, it causes the feelings of mental sluggishness, decreased capacity for activity and feelings of fatigue. It also leads to a decrease in the operation of some of the major body functions, as the body would be busy trying to look for ways to look for nutrients to maintain its operation.

While the main intention for starving yourself may be to lose weight, you may end up causing other great impacts on your body. For instance, this leads to low production of hormones that can cause lower sex drive and fertility rate in women who have passed the puberty age; there may be an abrupt stop in menstruation while in men the production of sperms may be inactive. In children who have not passed the puberty age, it leads to permanent lose in fertility. In addition, starvation can make the brain to lack concentration, which can as well facilitate the development of increased anxiety, fatigue or even depression.

The continuity in this problem can also make your brain to decrease in performance something that in most cases would leave you in a state of torpor and fatigue. Bearing in mind the impacts of starvation, I recommend obesity victims to rather consider other methods of weight loss.

Increase The Intake Of Proteins

Increasing the intake of proteins and reducing the intake of carbohydrates can boost the success of your weight loss program. Normally, proteins are known to contain various amino acids among which are leucine and leptin. The leucine component in proteins works effectively in reducing the levels of triglycerides in that it helps leptin to easily get into your brain, which means you would feel full after consuming a few calories. It is known that when leptin gets into the brain, it reduces leptin resistance, which ensures metabolism is increased. If you are among the many people like me who find it hard to lower consumption of calories, eating proteins can boost your success greatly.

The great thing with reduced intake of food is that it encourages your body to break down some of the stored fats, which prevents the body from converting muscle proteins to fuel that can preserve muscle mass. Increasing the intake of proteins also wakes up the liver giving it something to do which means an increase in your metabolic rate. Considering that the liver the largest metabolic factory, boosting its functioning enables it to burn more calories. In addition, most of the enzymes, hormones and neurotransmitters that boost the weight loss progress require the use of special proteins that are mostly made by the liver.

Add Fruits And Vegetables To Your Diet

Fruits and vegetables are classified under the class of vitamins, which means they are natural foods that contain various minerals and chemicals. These foods contain low fat levels, calorie levels, less water retention, low sodium levels, and high fiber, which enable them to fill the stomach quickly and increase vitality due to their high nutrient value. All these features in vegetables and fruits enable them to effectively control ones weight when taken in the right measurements. This is mostly because they are low in calories, which means one can eat lots of vegetables without consuming excess energy.

They are also rich in fiber, which ensure that you can eat small amounts and still feel satisfied. The vitamins and chemicals in vegetables also help the body to continue gaining more energy since they supply the suitable nutrients that are needed to boost the production of energy within the muscle cells. Since vegetables are low in sodium, they also help reduce the increased water gain in your body.

Considering that sodium occurs in form of all processed foods, it enables your body to hold water within the interstitial areas of the body, when it is taken in low quantities, it helps lower water weight. This way, including the intake of vegetables in the food you take has numerous advantages in your weight loss program.

Giving Your Kitchen A Makeover Is Also Ideal

You should also start changing your eating habits drastically. For instance, you need to get rid of all processed foods and any other garbage food that is known to thwart your weight loss efforts. You should not just remove it for the time you would be fighting obesity but for the rest of your life. You must also create some kind of enmity between you and such foods as this would ensure that you would never bother yourself to purchase it when you see it in the stores. After you are sure within yourself that you have eradicated such foods, you should then refill your kitchen with whole and fresh foods.

Depending on your financial ability, you can do this at once or do it slowly. When trying to get rig any junk food within your kitchen, you should make sure that you do it with moderation to avoid harming yourself. For instance, since it is hard to stop eating certain foods at once you can decide to be reducing the intake amount from time to time since this would help you quit it completely within a certain period.

Control Your Workouts

Always Be Responsible

From a personal experience, I have learnt that engaging on a self-controlled workout is cheap and effective if you remain faithful and genuine to your workout program but very tricky if you do not emphasize on these factors. As a result, while you may consider it better to use a self-controlled workout program to lose weight, joining a weight-loss program where a professional controls everything from the management of your attendance to the recording of your progression can have numerous benefits.

Even though it seems costly to hire a fitness trainer, using their services is guaranteed of positive results. One of the main reasons for having a professional is that you will get proper guidance on what you should be doing in order to attain full control of your weight problem. You can even start knowing more things about your body that you never knew depending on how frequently you interact with the trainer.

Considering that these professionals would have enough experience in offering these services, they would ensure that they offer the best. In addition, since you would meet with many other people who are on the same journey, you would get the morale to do your best.

Keep Records Of Your Initial Weight

When embarking on a workout program, it is essential to make sure that you know your weight status in order to determine what to do and how to do it to achieve your weight targets. This means the scale is an essential tool for the success of your plans. It is advisable to be taking down your weight and recording it once every week or month.

Being in a position to know your progress would enable you determine whether you need to make an improvement in the weight loss program as well as empowering you to keep exercising until you reach your set goals. However, it is not advisable to be weighing yourself each day since when the body burn calories, it does not show an immediate change on your physical size and weight that means taking measurements each day can discourage you. It is as well essential to be taking the measurements of your arms, neck, hips, chest, waist and thigh to determine where there is any change that has occurred within the days you have been working out.

When doing this, you should always keep in mind that in order to succeed in your workout program, your desire for success should be greater than your fear of failure as once you allow fear to drive you, the chances are that you would not make it.

Take Time To Set Up An Anchor

One best feature of a productive and successful workout program is the existence of an anchor. An anchor is a product or substance that keeps reminding people on their progression. I have seen people using different approaches to track performance. One of which I preferred most is the paper clip chain which is designed portable and flexible enough.

With this anchor, you can be carrying it anywhere from time to time to ensure that you can always tell how well you are performing. An anchor actually gives someone the option to know the exact number of pounds he or she has lost between two measurement dates.

However, when taking this weight loss program, you should always make sure that you are observant on each step you take, as this would boost your likelihood of success. Try to avoid not recording your progress since you can easily forget making it possible that you may not understand the specific amount of weight lost.

Initiate A Manageable Workout Routine

Everybody knows that a good workout program is not just a matter of waking up one morning and deciding to be making few trips around your backyard. It entails the need for devotion and self-empowerment.

Therefore, if you want to succeed in your quest towards a sustainable workout program, it is advisable to make sure that you take the right measures and steps. For instance, start with easy routines to make you feel comfortable as you move up to the harder, more strenuous ones. You should also make sure that you are not engaging in a project that would make you feel uncomfortable and not happy with yourself. It should be made in such a way that it will help you achieve your goals of losing as many calories as possible. For instance, there would be no need to waste your time and energy settling for a workout program that would require you to spend more time than you can dedicate.

Be Passionate On Your Workout

Thinking Outside The Gym Is Too Great To Boost Your Success

As from studies, saving at least 40 minutes each day to participate in cardiovascular exercise sessions of strong training is ideal to help someone fight obesity. However, embarking on lifestyle-based activities such as standing while taking on a phone, walking the rest of the way to and from work and getting off a bus or train few meters before the stopping point can be a great alternative.

You can as well decide to engage in active hobbies such as taking dance lessons instead of photography lessons or bowling instead of going to watch movies. This is mostly because when dancing, you will not only enjoy listening to the songs of your favorite singers but also enjoy the benefits that come with burning some calories in the process.

Participating in basic things such as driving cars, washing dishes, using elevators and washing machines can help people burn a few calories per day. As a result, boosting your workout program with a non-exercise fun activity like participating in the above given programs can enable one boost their chances of achieving their weight lose goals.

You Must Also Be Flexible Enough To Adapt To Changes

Even though there are many lifestyle changes that happen each day that are assumed to help you achieve your weight loss dreams, your preferences play a great role in testing you.

For instance, consider a situation when you will work until late hours such that you will not have enough time to get to the gym or a situation when you will be stuck in traffic making you to miss your fitness class. Such instances clearly show that workout is not easy; however, you shouldn't let this distract you from the goal of attaining your desired weight especially when you already have a program that you are following.

Flexibility is the only factor or formula that can help you solve the problems that come naturally to affect your workout plan. For instance, you should always consider carrying some workout shoes in your car to ensure that if you run late for the gym, you can pass by the park and take a quick walk.

You should also carry food with you to ensure that if you are stuck in traffic, you would easily have a snack before you set on for your workout. In most cases, many people skip workouts just because of minor things that if controlled, someone may have achieved something else beneficial as the scheduled workout.

Maximize Every Second To Get Fit

In a weight loss program, every single step you take counts and can enable you to either achieve your weight loss target or fail to realize that you were taking a weight loss program. You should thus be smart on your doings and make sure that you can make the most out the little time you would have for workout. For instance, it is wise to try to fit in small exercise bouts whenever you have time for doing it such as chewing gum when watching television, doing jumping jacks or dancing when washing dishes.

This always enables your body to burn calories and save you from mindless munching when watching television or doing any other stuff. You can also utilize the little time you have when going to work to run and take some exercise rather that crawling slowly since this may contribute to your weight problem. Before going to bed, you can also spent some few minutes to take press ups as this would boost your weight loss success.

After waking up in the morning, rather than going for a shower directly, you can also run around your house severally. This way, you would be using the little time you have to make your weight loss program effective.

Know Your Limits

Try To Make Friends With People Who Have Positive Ideas

Initiating a workout program to cut down those extra calories is one of the most important decisions one can make in life. As a result, trying to engage yourself in a workout is more than just having negative-minded friends who keep advising you to quit your workout. It is known that the kind of people you live with are one of the main determinants of the kind of person you can be hence living with people who advise you to quit exercises can affect your plans greatly.

As such, once you discover that your friends do not give a helping hand to boost your new lifestyle, it would be better to get new friends. For instance, if your plans are to reduce the intake of alcohol and bad food, but the friends you have want you to keep on eating the foods you want to quit and drinking alcohol, it would be a great solution to bid them a farewell.

With the many challenges associated with the journey to lose weight, surrounding yourself with positive friends can be the only thing you will need by then. You should make sure that the friends you have do not influence you negatively since this would assure that you are on the right way to your weight lose program.

Make Your Way Out Of Alcohol Consumption

When looking to fight obesity, you should make alcohol your first-class enemy even if it has been your best drink. I don't personally hate alcohol nor do I hate anyone who takes it but looking at what researchers have found, making alcohol your best friend when participating on a weight loss program is the same as spraying your plants with pesticides and insecticides but leave the weeds that attract the insects and pests around the plants.

This is because when we talk of weight loss, it means we want to burn more calories than we are consuming. However, as most studies show, when someone drinks alcohol, it would be broken into acetate, a dietary that the body burns first before any other calorie that is consumed or stored in the body. Consequently, when you drink alcohol and consume more calories most commonly, your body would store the fat from such diets since it would be obtaining its energy from the acetate. Alcohol is also known to inhibit lipid oxidation, which means once you drink it, your body would not be able to burn stored fats or the fats from the food you eat.

Some scientific proves also claim that when someone drinks excess alcohol, they end up passing a threshold after which a certain portion of the alcohol calories are free which not only make you fat but also facilitate the development of liver problems like fatty liver disease which can further develop to cirrhosis and finally death. Therefore, when you initiate a weight lose workout, it would be essential to make sure that you reduce or stop the intake of any alcoholic drinks.

Avoid Eating Out Especially From Hotels

I thought eating out could make me feel more relaxed and reduce my spending, but after I realized the harm I was causing to my body, I decided to keep this habit as low as possible; there are days you definitely want to spoil yourself! First, after I did the evaluation on the foods I was ordering from hotels I realized that in all the occasions it was just once after a week I could leave the plate un-cleared, meaning in most cases I always overfed myself just because I wanted to make the most use of my money.

In addition, each time I visited a hotel I used to make sure that I did not just eat the food alone but added few other drinks that I found they always boosted my appetite other than making it lower. This has since subsided especially when I eat my own home cooked food since I can portion my food for every meal and keep any that I don't need now for later consumption. Keep the frequency of emotional eating as low as possible since this can actually make you eat more than necessary.

Limiting The Intake Of Liquid Calories Is Also A Solution

Our bodies are designed in such a way that they would not register liquid calories the same way they do to the calories from solid foods meaning it is usually easier for us to eat more calories when drinking than when eating foods rich in calories. This is mostly because we do not chew liquid foods that cause a decrease in exocrine and endocrine that is produced when we eat solid foods. In addition, our stomachs empty liquid foods quicker than solid foods, which lead to weaker hunger signals hence making someone to eat more.

This means that if you take calories in form of liquids, high chances are that you might have a problem in succeeding in your weight loss program since you would always be consuming more calories than your desired amount. Personally, I advise people to keep their consumption of solid foods like sugar-sweetened drinks like tea, sport drinks and juice low. When you understand your needs and take on the idea of eating foods rich in calories rather than drinking foods rich in calories, you would boost your plan of fighting obesity.

Conclusion

We have come to the end of the book. Thank you for reading and congratulations for reading until the end.

I really hope that you have found the book educative on effective ways through which you can lose weight easily and keep it off for good. Now is your turn to implement everything you learned.

Now is your turn to take action!

My Other Books

[Binge Eating: Binge Eating Disorder Cure: Easy To Follow Tips For Eating Only What Your Body Needs](#)

[Lose Weight: Lose Weight Fast Naturally: How to Lose Weight Fast Without Having To Become a Gym Rat or Dieting Like a Maniac](#)

[Lose Weight: Lose Weight Permanently: Effective Strategies on How to Lose Weight Easily and Permanently](#)

[KETOGENIC DIET: Keto Diet Made Easy: Beginners Guide on How to Burn Fat Fast With the Keto Diet (Including 100+ Recipes That You Can Prepare Within 20 Minutes)- New Edition](#)

[KETOGENIC DIET: Ketogenic Diet Recipes That You Can Prepare Using 7 Ingredients and Less in Less Than 30 Minutes](#)

[Ketogenic Diet: Lose Weight Rapidly With Paleo Friendly Ketogenic Diet Recipes You Can Make Within 25 Minutes](#)